CONTENTS

INTRODUCTION

In the world of culinary delights and dietary considerations, the quest for healthier alternatives to traditional sweeteners has given rise to a remarkable natural treasure: monk fruit sweetener. As our understanding of the impacts of excessive sugar consumption on health continues to deepen, the search for a sweet solution that offers both indulgence and wellbeing becomes ever more crucial. Enter monk fruit sweetener, an intriguing and ancient fruit that has captured the attention of health-conscious individuals, culinary experts, and researchers alike. In this exploration, we delve into the origins, benefits, myths, and practical applications of monk fruit sweetener, uncovering its journey from the enigmatic realm of traditional medicine to the forefront of modern dietary choices. Embark with us on a journey through the history, science, and culinary artistry that shapes the narrative of monk fruit sweetener, a true testament to the harmonious fusion of nature's sweetness and human innovation.

CHAPTER ONE

Introduction to Monk Fruit Sweetener

Brief history and origin of monk fruit:

Monk fruit, scientifically known as Siraitia grosvenorii and also referred to as Luo Han Guo, has a rich history deeply rooted in Eastern cultures, particularly in China and Thailand. Its name alone conjures up a sense of mystique and ancient wisdom. The fruit's origin can be traced back to the Guilin region in southern China, where it has been cultivated for centuries. The plant belongs to the Cucurbitaceae family, which includes cucumbers, melons, and gourds, and its unique sweetening properties have made it a treasured ingredient in traditional medicine and cuisine.

In Chinese folklore, monk fruit is associated with the monks of the 13th century, who are believed to have introduced its use as a natural sweetener. They cultivated the fruit in the mist-covered mountains of Guilin and utilized it in herbal remedies and teas for its purported health benefits. The fruit's appeal extended beyond its sweetness; it was also recognized for its potential to balance the body's elements and alleviate ailments.

Monk fruit's journey from traditional medicine to modern sweetener:

1. Rediscovery of Monk Fruit's Sweetness:

For centuries, monk fruit remained a well-kept secret of the East, known only to those immersed in traditional Chinese medicine. However, the 20th century witnessed a turning point as the fruit's incredible sweetness caught the attention of Western researchers. In 1918, botanist Gilbert H. Stace discovered the plant during his travels in China and introduced it to the scientific community. The sweetness was attributed to unique compounds called mogrosides found in the fruit's extract.

2. Mogrosides and Sweetening Potential:

Mogrosides, specifically mogroside V, are the key compounds responsible for monk fruit's intense sweetness. These natural compounds are non-caloric and do not impact blood sugar levels, making them a promising alternative to traditional sugars for individuals with diabetes or those seeking to reduce sugar consumption. Mogrosides are estimated to be around 150 to 200 times sweeter than sucrose, the common table sugar.

3. Transition to the Modern Food Industry:

In the latter half of the 20th century, as concerns about health and sugar consumption escalated, the food industry began to search for healthier sweetening alternatives. Monk fruit's potential as a natural, zero-calorie sweetener started gaining traction. However, challenges arose due to the fruit's perishability and limited cultivation areas. This led to the development of monk fruit extracts and powders, making it easier to incorporate the sweetener into various food and beverage products.

4. Regulatory Approvals and Commercialization:

The path from traditional herbal remedy to mainstream sweetener required rigorous scientific studies and regulatory approvals. In the early 2000s, monk fruit extracts received Generally Recognized as Safe (GRAS) status from regulatory bodies such as the U.S. Food and Drug Administration (FDA). This green light paved the way for monk fruit to emerge as a natural sweetening option in the global market. Major food and beverage companies began to incorporate monk fruit extracts into their products as a response to consumer demands for healthier alternatives.

5. Monk Fruit's Appeal and Challenges:

Monk fruit's journey from traditional medicine to modern sweetener was not without hurdles. While its exceptional sweetness and potential health benefits intrigued consumers, some challenges emerged. The relatively higher cost of monk fruit extracts compared to traditional sweeteners posed a financial obstacle for widespread adoption. Additionally, formulating with monk fruit required overcoming technical issues related to taste, solubility, and stability in various food and beverage applications.

6. The Rise of Monk Fruit Sweeteners:

Despite the challenges, monk fruit sweeteners have carved out a niche in the market as a viable natural alternative to sugar and artificial sweeteners. They are found in a range of products, including beverages, desserts, baked goods, and even condiments. Health-conscious consumers have welcomed monk fruit sweeteners due to their low-calorie and low-glycemic nature, aligning with trends toward cleaner eating.

7. Looking Ahead: Innovation and Potential:

As consumer preferences evolve and health concerns continue to drive food trends, monk fruit sweeteners stand poised for further growth and innovation. Ongoing research is exploring the potential applications of monk fruit in dietary supplements, pharmaceuticals, and beyond. Continued advancements in extraction techniques, taste optimization, and cost reduction could expand the reach of monk fruit as a versatile sweetening solution.

In conclusion, the journey of monk fruit from its historical roots in traditional Chinese medicine to its current status as a sought-after natural sweetener is a testament to the interplay between ancient wisdom and modern scientific exploration. The rediscovery of monk fruit's unique sweetness, the isolation of its potent mogroside compounds, and its transformation into a commercial sweetening option highlight the intricate relationship between nature's gifts and human ingenuity. As monk fruit continues to captivate taste buds and redefine sweetness, it reminds us that the journey from obscurity to prominence is marked by a delicate balance of tradition and innovation.

CHAPTER TWO

Understanding Monk Fruit

Botanical features and growth conditions of monk fruit:

Monk fruit, scientifically known as Siraitia grosvenorii, is a perennial vine belonging to the Cucurbitaceae family. This family also includes cucumbers, melons, and gourds. The plant has distinct features that contribute to its growth and fruit production. Monk fruit vines can reach lengths of up to 5 meters and are characterized by their heart-shaped leaves with serrated edges. The vines produce tendrils that allow them to climb and twine around support structures.

The monk fruit's unique fruit, also called a "monk fruit" or "Buddha fruit," is small and round, measuring around 5 to 7 centimeters in diameter. It has a hard, green outer shell with light green markings and turns brown upon ripening. The inner flesh contains the fruit's seeds and the sweetening compounds known as mogrosides. Monk fruit plants thrive in subtropical climates with well-drained soil, plenty of sunlight, and adequate moisture. The Guilin region in southern China is the primary cultivation area due to its suitable climate and terrain.

Nutritional profile and natural compounds found in monk fruit:

Monk fruit is renowned for its exceptional sweetness without the calories and blood sugar impacts associated with traditional sugars. Its nutritional profile is notable for being low in calories, carbohydrates, and sugars. The majority of monk fruit's sweetness comes from its unique natural compounds known as mogrosides. These mogrosides are classified into different types (V, VI, and VII), with mogroside V being the most abundant and sweetest.

Beyond mogrosides, monk fruit also contains vitamins, minerals, and antioxidants. While its levels of these nutrients are not as high as in some other fruits, the presence of antioxidants like vitamin C and vitamin E contributes to the fruit's potential health benefits. Monk fruit's antioxidant properties are attributed to its ability to scavenge free radicals and reduce oxidative stress.

Comparison with other natural and artificial sweeteners:

Monk Fruit vs. Traditional Sugars:

Monk fruit's sweetness is primarily derived from mogrosides, which are compounds that do not raise blood sugar levels, making them suitable for individuals with diabetes or those watching their sugar intake. In contrast, traditional sugars like sucrose and high-fructose corn syrup can cause rapid spikes in blood glucose levels, leading to potential health issues such as insulin resistance and weight gain.

Monk Fruit vs. Stevia:

Stevia, another natural sweetener, is extracted from the leaves of the Stevia rebaudiana plant. Both monk fruit and stevia offer sweetness without the calories of sugar, but they have distinct flavor profiles. While stevia can sometimes have a slightly bitter aftertaste, monk fruit is often described as having a cleaner, more neutral taste. The choice between the two may come down to personal preference and the specific application in which they are used.

Monk Fruit vs. Artificial Sweeteners:

Artificial sweeteners like aspartame, saccharin, and sucralose are synthetic compounds used as sugar substitutes. Unlike monk fruit, these sweeteners are not derived from natural sources. Some artificial sweeteners have been linked to controversial health concerns, leading many consumers to seek natural alternatives. Monk fruit, being a natural sweetener with a long history of traditional use, provides a compelling option for those seeking sweetness without synthetic additives.

Monk Fruit vs. Honey and Agave Nectar:

Honey and agave nectar are often considered healthier alternatives to refined sugars due to their natural origins. However, they still contain significant amounts of fructose and calories. Monk fruit, on the other hand, has a negligible calorie and carbohydrate content, making it a desirable option for those looking to reduce calorie intake and minimize the impact on blood sugar levels.

Monk Fruit and the Clean Label Trend:

As consumers become more conscious of the ingredients in their food and beverages, the clean label trend has gained momentum. Monk fruit fits well within this trend due to its natural origin and minimal processing. Its sweetness allows manufacturers to reduce or eliminate added sugars without compromising on taste. This aligns with the preferences of health-conscious consumers who are actively seeking out products with simpler, recognizable ingredients.

In conclusion, monk fruit's botanical features, growth conditions, nutritional profile, and unique natural compounds make it a standout option among sweeteners. Its journey from a traditional Chinese remedy to a modern, commercially viable sweetening solution underscores its significance in the evolving landscape of food and beverage innovation. When compared to other sweeteners, monk fruit's ability to provide sweetness without calories, carbohydrates, and blood sugar impacts makes it a remarkable and versatile choice for individuals striving to make healthier dietary choices.

CHAPTER THREE

*The Science Behind Monk
Fruit Sweetness*

Exploring the key compound responsible for sweetness: mogrosides:

At the heart of monk fruit's remarkable sweetness lies a group of natural compounds known as mogrosides. These compounds are glycosides, meaning they consist of a sugar molecule attached to a non-sugar molecule. In the case of mogrosides, the non-sugar molecule is responsible for the intense sweetness, while the attached sugar portion contributes to the overall structure. Mogroside V, the most abundant and sweetest of the mogrosides, is responsible for monk fruit's unique flavor profile.

Mogrosides are non-caloric and do not raise blood sugar levels, making them an attractive alternative to traditional sugars. They have a sweetness that can be up to 200 times that of sucrose (table sugar), which means only a small amount is needed to achieve the desired level of sweetness in foods and beverages. The intriguing aspect of mogrosides is that despite their incredible sweetness, they do not leave a lingering aftertaste like some artificial sweeteners. This makes monk fruit sweetener a sought-after option for those seeking a clean and natural taste.

How mogrosides are extracted and processed into monk

fruit sweetener:

The process of turning monk fruit into a sweetening agent involves extracting the mogrosides from the fruit and transforming them into a usable form. Here's a simplified breakdown of the extraction and processing steps:

- Harvesting: Monk fruit is harvested when ripe, typically from late summer to early autumn. The fruit is carefully collected, as its thin skin can be easily damaged.
- Extraction: The first step is to extract the mogrosides from the monk fruit. This is often done by crushing or pressing the fruit to release its juice. The juice contains the mogrosides, as well as other components like water and pulp.
- Filtration: The extracted juice undergoes filtration to remove any solid particles or impurities. This results in a clearer liquid.
- Concentration: The filtered juice is then concentrated to increase the concentration of mogrosides. This can involve methods such as evaporation or membrane filtration.
- Purification: Further purification processes are employed to isolate mogroside compounds from other components. Chromatography, a technique used to separate and purify substances, is often utilized for this step.
- Drying: The purified mogrosides are dried to remove any remaining moisture, resulting in a powdered form that is easier to handle and incorporate into various products.
- Blending and Formulation: Depending on the intended use, the powdered monk fruit sweetener

can be blended with other ingredients or carriers to achieve the desired texture and sweetness level. This makes it suitable for applications such as beverages, baked goods, and sauces.

Understanding the sweetness potency and flavor profile:

Mogrosides' intense sweetness potency is a standout feature that sets monk fruit sweetener apart from other natural and artificial sweeteners. While the exact sweetness level can vary based on factors like the specific type of mogroside and the concentration used, it's generally accepted that mogroside V, the predominant component, is approximately 150 to 200 times sweeter than sucrose.

In terms of flavor profile, monk fruit sweetener is celebrated for its clean and neutral taste. Unlike some artificial sweeteners that can leave a bitter or metallic aftertaste, monk fruit sweetener doesn't carry such drawbacks. This makes it an ideal choice for enhancing the sweetness of foods and beverages without compromising their overall flavor. The absence of an aftertaste contributes to the natural and satisfying sensory experience monk fruit sweetener offers.

It's worth noting that while monk fruit sweetener excels in taste, its texture and behavior in certain culinary applications might differ slightly from traditional sugars due to its unique properties. For instance, in baked goods, the absence of sugar's bulk and moisture-retaining properties might require recipe adjustments. Nonetheless, manufacturers and chefs have been experimenting and innovating to ensure the successful integration of monk fruit sweetener in various recipes without compromising on taste or quality.

In conclusion, the exploration of mogrosides as the key compounds responsible for monk fruit's sweetness reveals the intricate nature of this natural sweetener. The extraction and processing of mogrosides from monk fruit into a usable sweetening agent showcases the fusion of traditional wisdom with modern technology. As consumers continue to seek healthier and more natural alternatives to sugars and artificial sweeteners, the potency of mogrosides, combined with their neutral flavor profile, positions monk fruit sweetener as a frontrunner in the evolving landscape of sweetening solutions.

CHAPTER FOUR

Health Benefits of Monk Fruit Sweetener

Zero-calorie nature and its impact on weight management:

Monk fruit sweetener's zero-calorie characteristic has garnered significant attention from individuals striving to manage their weight. Unlike traditional sugars that contribute calories without offering substantial nutritional benefits, monk fruit sweetener provides sweetness without the caloric load. This makes it an attractive option for those looking to reduce overall calorie intake and maintain a healthy weight.

By substituting high-calorie sugars with monk fruit sweetener in foods and beverages, individuals can enjoy the sensation of sweetness without the corresponding increase in energy consumption. This reduction in caloric intake is particularly beneficial for weight management and weight loss goals. Incorporating monk fruit sweetener into one's diet can aid in creating a calorie deficit, which is a fundamental principle in achieving weight loss.

Glycemic index and suitability for diabetics and those monitoring blood sugar:

The glycemic index (GI) is a measure that indicates

how quickly a carbohydrate-containing food raises blood glucose levels. Foods with a high GI can lead to rapid spikes and crashes in blood sugar levels, while those with a low GI have a more gradual impact. Monk fruit sweetener has a negligible effect on blood sugar due to its minimal carbohydrate content and the fact that its sweetness comes from non-caloric mogrosides.

This quality makes monk fruit sweetener an excellent choice for individuals with diabetes or those who need to monitor their blood sugar levels. Unlike traditional sugars that can cause blood sugar spikes, monk fruit sweetener can be safely included in the diets of people managing diabetes without compromising their blood glucose control.

Antioxidant properties and potential health-boosting effects:

In addition to its role as a natural sweetener, monk fruit boasts antioxidant properties that have piqued the interest of researchers and health enthusiasts alike. Antioxidants play a crucial role in combating oxidative stress and reducing damage caused by free radicals in the body. Monk fruit contains antioxidants such as vitamin C and vitamin E, albeit in modest amounts compared to certain other fruits and vegetables.

While the antioxidant levels in monk fruit may not be as high as in berries or leafy greens, the presence of these compounds suggests potential health-boosting effects. Antioxidants are known to support overall health and wellness, contributing to the prevention of chronic diseases such as heart disease, certain cancers, and neurodegenerative conditions. Including monk fruit sweetener in one's diet could provide an additional source of antioxidants to complement a balanced and nutrient-rich eating plan.

Summing up the health benefits and considerations:

Monk fruit sweetener's zero-calorie nature and low glycemic impact make it a suitable choice for individuals focused on weight management and blood sugar control. Its versatility as a sugar substitute allows for a more flexible approach to sweetness in foods and beverages without the drawbacks of excess calories and blood sugar fluctuations. Moreover, the potential antioxidant properties of monk fruit sweetener add a layer of potential health benefits beyond its role as a sugar alternative.

However, while monk fruit sweetener offers several advantages, it's important to remember that moderation is key. While it doesn't raise blood sugar, individuals should be mindful of portion sizes and overall dietary choices. Also, as with any sweetener, it's advisable to consult with a healthcare professional, especially for individuals with specific health conditions or dietary concerns.

In conclusion, monk fruit sweetener's combination of zero-calorie sweetness, low glycemic impact, and potential antioxidant properties positions it as a valuable addition to the arsenal of individuals pursuing a healthier lifestyle. Its suitability for weight management, blood sugar control, and potential health benefits make it a preferred option for those seeking to balance their desire for sweetness with their health objectives.

CHAPTER FIVE

Monk Fruit Sweetener
in the Kitchen

Culinary uses and applications in cooking and baking:

Monk fruit sweetener's versatility extends beyond being a mere sugar substitute. It has found its way into a wide range of culinary creations, from beverages and desserts to savory dishes. Here are some of its notable applications:

- Beverages: Monk fruit sweetener dissolves easily in liquids, making it a popular choice for sweetening beverages like teas, coffees, smoothies, and even cocktails.
- Baking: Monk fruit sweetener can be used in baking, but some adjustments are often required due to its lack of bulk and moisture-holding properties. It's ideal for recipes like cookies, cakes, and muffins where sugar's primary function is sweetness.
- Sauces and Dressings: Monk fruit sweetener can be used in sauces, dressings, and marinades to balance flavors and add a touch of sweetness.
- Yogurts and Dairy Alternatives: It can be blended into yogurt, dairy alternatives, or even cottage cheese for a naturally sweetened experience.
- Jams and Spreads: Monk fruit sweetener can be used to sweeten homemade jams, jellies, and nut

butters.

- Frozen Desserts: It can be used in recipes for ice creams, sorbets, and frozen yogurts.

Conversion guidelines for substituting traditional sugar with monk fruit sweetener:

Substituting monk fruit sweetener for traditional sugar requires some adjustment due to the unique characteristics of each sweetener. Here are general guidelines to help with conversions:

- Sweetness Intensity: Monk fruit sweetener is much sweeter than sugar, so you'll need significantly less. A common guideline is to use about 1/4 to 1/2 teaspoon of monk fruit sweetener per 1 teaspoon of sugar.
- Bulk and Texture: Monk fruit sweetener lacks the bulk and moisture provided by sugar. In baking, consider adding a binding agent like applesauce or yogurt to help maintain the desired texture.
- Liquid Adjustments: Monk fruit sweetener can absorb more liquid than sugar. Adjust the liquid content in your recipe accordingly.
- Baking Powder: Since sugar contributes to the activation of baking powder, consider using a slightly larger amount of baking powder when using monk fruit sweetener to ensure proper rise.
- Recipe Testing: Given the unique properties of monk fruit sweetener, some experimentation might be necessary to achieve the desired results in your recipes. Start with small adjustments and gradually fine-tune the proportions.

Flavor nuances and adjustments for achieving desired taste profiles:

Monk fruit sweetener's neutral flavor profile is a great asset when it comes to achieving the desired taste in recipes. However, depending on the specific application, you might want to tweak the flavor profile to suit your preferences. Here are some considerations:

- Balancing Bitterness: Monk fruit sweetener can sometimes have a slightly bitter aftertaste. To counteract this, consider using flavor enhancers like vanilla extract, almond extract, or a pinch of salt to balance the flavors.
- Combining Sweeteners: If you prefer to avoid any potential bitterness, you can blend monk fruit sweetener with other natural sweeteners like erythritol or stevia. These combinations can provide a more well-rounded sweetness profile.
- Citrus and Acidity: In recipes that involve citrus fruits or other acidic ingredients, monk fruit sweetener can complement the acidity by adding sweetness without overpowering the natural flavors.
- Herbs and Spices: Monk fruit sweetener pairs well with various herbs and spices, allowing you to create complex flavor profiles in both sweet and savory dishes.
- Gradual Adaptation: If you're transitioning from traditional sugar to monk fruit sweetener, your taste buds might need time to adjust. Gradually reducing the amount of sugar in your recipes and increasing the amount of monk fruit sweetener can help ease the transition.

In summary, monk fruit sweetener's adaptability makes it a valuable ingredient in a variety of culinary creations. Its intense sweetness, negligible caloric impact, and neutral flavor open up opportunities to enjoy sweetness in a health-conscious manner. While conversions and adjustments might be needed, experimenting with monk fruit sweetener in different recipes can lead to delightful results that cater to individual taste preferences.

CHAPTER SIX

Addressing Common Concerns

Safety and potential side effects of consuming monk fruit sweetener:

Monk fruit sweetener is generally considered safe for consumption when used in moderation. It has been extensively studied, and no serious adverse effects have been reported. However, like any food or additive, there are a few considerations to keep in mind:

- Gastrointestinal Distress: Consuming large amounts of monk fruit sweetener, especially in concentrated forms, may lead to gastrointestinal discomfort such as bloating, gas, or diarrhea. Moderation is key to avoiding these potential side effects.
- Allergic Reactions: While rare, some individuals might be sensitive or allergic to certain components of monk fruit sweetener. If you experience any allergic reactions such as itching, hives, or difficulty breathing after consuming monk fruit products, seek medical attention.
- Laxative Effect: Like many sugar alcohols, monk fruit sweetener may have a mild laxative effect if consumed in excessive quantities. This is more likely to occur when consuming products containing other sweeteners like erythritol.

It's important to note that individual responses can vary, and what works well for one person may not be the same for another. Consulting with a healthcare professional before making any significant dietary changes is always advisable, especially for individuals with pre-existing medical conditions or sensitivities.

Allergies and sensitivities associated with monk fruit:

True allergies to monk fruit are extremely rare. The compounds responsible for monk fruit's sweetness, mogrosides, are generally not associated with common food allergies. However, some individuals might have sensitivities to specific components present in monk fruit products, such as fillers or additives used in blends.

If you suspect an allergic reaction to monk fruit, discontinue its use and consult with a healthcare professional. In cases of severe allergies or sensitivities, it's recommended to perform a patch test or allergy testing before introducing monk fruit products into your diet.

Regulatory approvals and guidelines across different countries:

Monk fruit sweetener has gained regulatory approval as a food additive in various countries. However, regulations can vary, and it's essential to understand the specific guidelines in your region. As of my last knowledge update in September 2021, here are a few examples of regulatory approvals:

- United States (FDA): Monk fruit extract is generally recognized as safe (GRAS) when used as a food additive. The FDA has established guidelines for its use in different food categories.

- European Union (EU): Monk fruit sweetener is approved for use as a food additive in the EU under specific conditions. It's assigned a "E number," which signifies its approval for use within the EU.
- Australia and New Zealand: Monk fruit extract has been approved for use as a food additive in these countries, subject to specified conditions and usage levels.

It's important to stay updated on the latest regulatory information, as guidelines may evolve over time. When using monk fruit sweetener, ensure that you're selecting products that comply with local regulations and guidelines for safe consumption.

In conclusion, monk fruit sweetener is generally safe for consumption and has been approved for use as a food additive in various countries. While allergies and sensitivities are rare, individuals should be mindful of potential side effects and consult healthcare professionals if needed. Regulatory approvals vary by region, so staying informed about guidelines specific to your country is crucial when incorporating monk fruit sweetener into your diet.

CHAPTER SEVEN

Monk Fruit Sweetener in Personal Wellness

Incorporating monk fruit sweetener into various diets (keto, paleo, etc.):

Monk fruit sweetener's low-calorie and low-carbohydrate nature makes it a valuable addition to various diets that prioritize reduced sugar and carbohydrate intake. Here's how it can be incorporated into specific diets:

- Keto Diet: The ketogenic diet emphasizes high fat, low carbohydrate intake to induce ketosis. Monk fruit sweetener is keto-friendly due to its negligible impact on blood sugar and carbohydrate levels. It can be used to sweeten beverages, desserts, and even savory dishes without compromising ketosis.
- Paleo Diet: The paleo diet focuses on whole, unprocessed foods similar to those consumed by our ancestors. Monk fruit sweetener, being a natural extract, aligns well with the paleo philosophy. It can be used in moderation to add sweetness to paleo-friendly treats like baked goods and sauces.
- Low-Carb Diet: Monk fruit sweetener is a valuable tool for those following a low-carb diet, as it allows for the enjoyment of sweet flavors without

the carb content of sugar. It can be used creatively in a range of dishes while keeping carbohydrate intake in check.

- Diabetic-Friendly Diet: Monk fruit sweetener's lack of impact on blood sugar levels makes it an excellent choice for individuals with diabetes. It can be used to sweeten foods and beverages without causing spikes in blood glucose.
- Mindful Eating: Regardless of the specific diet, monk fruit sweetener supports mindful eating by providing a way to enjoy sweetness without the potential negative effects of traditional sugars. It allows individuals to savor flavors and satisfy cravings while maintaining a health-conscious approach to eating.

Role in reducing overall sugar intake and fostering mindful eating habits:

Monk fruit sweetener plays a pivotal role in reducing overall sugar intake, which is a central focus for health-conscious individuals. By using monk fruit sweetener instead of traditional sugars, individuals can enjoy sweetness with a lower calorie and carbohydrate burden. This is particularly important considering the excessive sugar consumption associated with many modern diets.

Fostering mindful eating habits involves being attuned to one's body, savoring flavors, and recognizing satiety cues. Monk fruit sweetener supports mindful eating by allowing individuals to experience the pleasure of sweetness without the potential downsides of excess sugar. It enables people to enjoy treats in moderation, appreciating the flavors and textures without overindulging.

Recipes and strategies for creating low-sugar, monk fruit-sweetened treats:

Creating low-sugar treats using monk fruit sweetener is a delightful way to enjoy sweetness while minimizing the impact on blood sugar and calorie intake. Here are some recipe ideas and strategies:

- Baking: Transform classic baking recipes into low-sugar versions by substituting monk fruit sweetener for sugar. Start with recipes that don't rely heavily on sugar's structure, such as cookies, brownies, and muffins. Keep in mind that adjustments might be needed for texture and moisture.
- Fruit Desserts: Combine monk fruit sweetener with fresh or cooked fruits to create delicious desserts with natural sweetness. For example, make a fruit salad with a touch of monk fruit sweetener or bake fruit crisps.
- Frozen Treats: Whip up low-sugar ice creams, popsicles, and frozen yogurt using monk fruit sweetener. Blend it with ingredients like coconut milk, nut butters, and fruits for creamy and satisfying treats.
- Beverages: Sweeten beverages like teas, lemonades, and smoothies with monk fruit sweetener. Adjust the amount to achieve your preferred level of sweetness.
- Sauces and Dressings: Add monk fruit sweetener to homemade sauces, dressings, and marinades to balance flavors and provide a touch of sweetness.
- No-Bake Treats: Create no-bake energy bites, protein bars, and truffles using monk fruit

sweetener for a guilt-free sweet fix.

When using monk fruit sweetener in recipes, consider starting with existing recipes that you enjoy and gradually making adjustments to fit your taste preferences. Keep in mind that monk fruit sweetener is much sweeter than sugar, so a little goes a long way. As you experiment and explore, you'll discover delightful ways to create low-sugar treats that align with your dietary goals and mindful eating approach.

CHAPTER EIGHT

Monk Fruit Sweetener and the Food Industry
Monk fruit sweetener as an ingredient in commercial food and beverage products:

Monk fruit sweetener has transitioned from a niche natural sweetener to a sought-after ingredient in the formulation of commercial food and beverage products. Its unique combination of zero-calorie sweetness and low glycemic impact has led to its incorporation into a wide range of products, including:

- Beverages: From carbonated drinks to flavored waters and energy drinks, monk fruit sweetener provides a healthier way to add sweetness without the high sugar content.
- Desserts: Ice creams, yogurts, and puddings benefit from monk fruit sweetener's ability to enhance sweetness without contributing to excessive calories.
- Bakery Goods: Manufacturers can create low-sugar or sugar-free baked goods that cater to health-conscious consumers and those with dietary restrictions.
- Snacks: Bars, protein snacks, and trail mixes can be sweetened with monk fruit to meet the growing demand for nutritious, low-sugar options.
- Condiments: Sauces, dressings, and spreads can

be reformulated to include monk fruit sweetener, appealing to consumers who want to reduce sugar in savory applications.

Market trends and consumer demand for healthier alternatives:

The global shift toward healthier lifestyles has propelled the demand for natural, low-calorie sweeteners like monk fruit. Key market trends and consumer demands driving the adoption of monk fruit sweetener include:

- Health-Conscious Consumers: As consumers become more health-conscious and seek to reduce sugar intake, they are actively seeking products that offer sweetness without the drawbacks of traditional sugars.
- Diabetes and Blood Sugar Management: The rise in diabetes cases and a growing interest in managing blood sugar levels have prompted consumers to explore sugar alternatives that have minimal impact on glucose.
- Clean Label Movement: Consumers are increasingly scrutinizing ingredient labels, favoring products with simple, recognizable ingredients. Monk fruit's natural origin aligns with the clean label trend.
- Weight Management: Those aiming to manage or lose weight are drawn to monk fruit's ability to provide sweetness without contributing to caloric intake.
- Plant-Based and Paleo Diets: The popularity of plant-based and paleo diets has boosted the demand for natural sweeteners that align with

these dietary preferences.

Challenges and opportunities for manufacturers using monk fruit sweetener:

While monk fruit sweetener offers numerous benefits, manufacturers also face challenges and opportunities as they incorporate it into their products:

Challenges:

- Cost: Monk fruit sweetener can be more expensive than other sweeteners, impacting production costs. However, advancements in extraction methods and increased demand may drive cost reduction over time.
- Formulation and Texture: Monk fruit's lack of bulk and moisture-retaining properties can pose challenges in certain applications, especially in baking. Manufacturers need to adjust formulations to achieve desired textures.
- Taste and Flavor: While monk fruit sweetener has a clean taste, it might require some flavor adjustments to match the sweetness profile of sugar and achieve desired taste perceptions.

Opportunities:

- Product Innovation: Manufacturers can innovate by creating new products or reformulating existing ones to cater to health-conscious consumers seeking low-sugar options.
- Clean Label Appeal: Incorporating monk fruit sweetener aligns with the clean label movement, providing manufacturers an opportunity to

attract consumers seeking transparency and natural ingredients.

- Health Claims: Manufacturers can capitalize on monk fruit's potential health benefits, such as its low glycemic impact and antioxidant properties, by incorporating relevant claims on packaging.
- Differentiated Offerings: As monk fruit sweetener gains popularity, products containing it can stand out in a crowded market, offering consumers a unique and healthier choice.

In conclusion, monk fruit sweetener's role as an ingredient in commercial food and beverage products is driven by evolving consumer preferences for healthier alternatives to traditional sugars. The market trends indicate a growing demand for products that offer sweetness without compromising on health and wellness. While challenges such as cost and formulation adjustments exist, manufacturers can leverage the opportunities presented by monk fruit sweetener's appeal, creating products that cater to the health-conscious and mindful consumer base.

CHAPTER NINE

Cultivation and Sustainability

Sustainable farming practices for monk fruit cultivation:

Sustainable farming practices are crucial to ensure the long-term viability of monk fruit cultivation while minimizing environmental impact. Some key sustainable practices for monk fruit cultivation include:

- Agroforestry: Intercropping monk fruit with other compatible plants can enhance biodiversity, improve soil health, and reduce the need for chemical inputs.
- Natural Pest Management: Implementing integrated pest management strategies, such as introducing beneficial insects and using natural predators, can help control pests without relying on synthetic chemicals.
- Soil Health: Using cover crops, crop rotation, and organic amendments can enhance soil fertility, structure, and water retention, promoting healthy plant growth.
- Water Conservation: Employing efficient irrigation systems and water management techniques helps conserve water resources and minimize waste.
- Organic Farming: Opting for organic farming practices reduces the use of synthetic fertilizers

and pesticides, resulting in healthier ecosystems and less chemical runoff.

- Community Engagement: Involving local communities in sustainable farming practices ensures cultural preservation and fosters responsible land use.

Environmental impact and benefits compared to other sweeteners:

Monk fruit sweetener has several environmental benefits compared to other sweeteners, particularly traditional sugars and some artificial sweeteners:

- Reduced Land Use: Monk fruit cultivation requires less land compared to crops like sugarcane, reducing deforestation and land conversion.
- Lower Water Usage: Monk fruit is often grown in regions with abundant rainfall, reducing the need for excessive irrigation that can deplete water resources.
- Lower Carbon Footprint: Monk fruit's efficiency in terms of land use, water, and resources contributes to a lower overall carbon footprint compared to other sweeteners.
- Biodiversity: Sustainable cultivation practices associated with monk fruit can support local ecosystems and promote biodiversity.
- Reduced Chemical Use: Organic and sustainable farming practices minimize chemical usage, decreasing the release of harmful pollutants into the environment.

Social and economic implications for communities

involved in monk fruit production:

Monk fruit cultivation can have positive social and economic impacts on communities involved in its production:

Employment Opportunities: Monk fruit cultivation and processing can provide employment opportunities, particularly in rural and economically marginalized areas.

- Income Generation: Cultivating monk fruit offers a potential source of income for farmers, improving their livelihoods and financial stability.
- Cultural Preservation: Sustainable farming practices can help preserve local traditions and indigenous knowledge related to monk fruit cultivation.
- Community Resilience: Monk fruit cultivation diversifies local economies, reducing dependency on single crops and enhancing community resilience.
- Access to Healthier Sweeteners: Monk fruit cultivation can contribute to local access to healthier sweeteners, promoting better dietary choices within communities.
- Fair Trade Practices: Implementing fair trade practices ensures that farmers receive fair compensation for their labor, promoting equitable distribution of benefits.

In conclusion, sustainable farming practices for monk fruit cultivation play a significant role in minimizing environmental impact, while monk fruit sweetener's benefits over other sweeteners contribute to a lower carbon footprint and greater biodiversity. Moreover, the social and economic implications of monk fruit production positively affect communities by providing employment, income, and cultural preservation opportunities. As the demand for healthier and sustainable sweeteners grows, responsible monk fruit cultivation can serve as a model for the coexistence of environmental stewardship and community well-being.

CHAPTER TEN

DIY Monk Fruit Sweetener Extraction

Step-by-step guide to extracting monk fruit sweetener at home:

Step 1: Harvest and Prepare Monk Fruit:

- Select ripe monk fruit with vibrant color and firm texture. Ripe monk fruit is sweeter.
- Wash the fruit thoroughly to remove any dirt or debris.

Step 2: Remove Seeds and Skin:

- Cut the monk fruit in half and scoop out the seeds with a spoon.
- Remove the skin using a knife or peeler. The skin is bitter and not used in the extraction process.

Step 3: Extract Mogrosides:

- Place the seedless and skinless monk fruit into a blender or food processor.
- Blend until the monk fruit turns into a smooth pulp.

Step 4: Strain the Pulp:

- Place a fine-mesh strainer or cheesecloth over a bowl.
- Pour the blended monk fruit pulp through the

strainer to separate the liquid from the solids.
- Gently press the pulp to extract as much liquid as possible.

Step 5: Heat and Reduce:

- Pour the strained monk fruit liquid into a saucepan.
- Heat the liquid over low heat, stirring occasionally, to evaporate excess water and concentrate the sweetness.
- Continue heating until the liquid has reduced by about half.

Step 6: Cool and Store:

- Allow the concentrated monk fruit liquid to cool.
- Transfer the sweetener to a clean, airtight container for storage.

Tools and equipment needed for the extraction process:

- Ripe monk fruit
- Knife and cutting board
- Blender or food processor
- Fine-mesh strainer or cheesecloth
- Bowl
- Saucepan
- Stirring utensil
- Clean, airtight container for storage

Tips for ensuring safety and quality in homemade monk fruit sweetener:

- Choose Ripe Fruit: Use fully ripe monk fruit for optimal sweetness and flavor.
- Clean Equipment: Ensure all tools and equipment

are clean and sanitized to prevent contamination.

- Avoid Skin and Seeds: Remove the skin and seeds, as they can contribute bitterness to the sweetener.
- Gentle Extraction: Strain the pulp gently to avoid forcing any bitterness from the skin and seeds into the sweetener.
- Low Heat: Use low heat when reducing the monk fruit liquid to prevent scorching or burning.
- Storing: Store the homemade sweetener in a clean, airtight container in the refrigerator. It should last for a few weeks.
- Experiment: Homemade sweetener might have variations in flavor and sweetness, so be prepared to experiment with the amount used in recipes.
- Safety: Be cautious when using heat and handling hot liquids. Use oven mitts or heat-resistant gloves as needed.

It's important to note that homemade monk fruit sweetener might not have the same potency or consistency as commercially produced versions. Commercial extraction processes are more advanced and can yield concentrated monk fruit sweeteners with precise sweetness levels. Additionally, the homemade process might not completely eliminate the bitter components, so taste-testing and adjusting are essential.

If you're looking for a more reliable and consistent monk fruit sweetener, it's recommended to purchase commercially available options from reputable brands. Homemade extraction is a fun experiment, but for regular use, commercially available monk fruit sweeteners are a safer and more convenient choice

CHAPTER ELEVEN

Future Outlook of Monk Fruit Sweetener

Ongoing research and potential discoveries related to monk fruit:

Ongoing research into monk fruit continues to unveil its potential benefits and applications. Some areas of research and potential discoveries include:

- Health Benefits: Researchers are exploring the potential health benefits of monk fruit beyond its sweetness. Studies are investigating its antioxidant properties, anti-inflammatory effects, and possible contributions to overall health and disease prevention.
- Pharmaceutical Uses: Some studies suggest that monk fruit's bioactive compounds, such as mogrosides, might have pharmaceutical applications, including in the development of new medications or supplements.
- Mogrosides and Health: Researchers are investigating how specific mogrosides interact with the body and exploring their impact on metabolic health, blood sugar regulation, and gut health.
- Culinary Applications: Researchers and chefs are working together to develop innovative culinary

applications for monk fruit in savory dishes, sauces, and complex flavor profiles.

Emerging applications and innovations in monk fruit-based products:

The versatility of monk fruit sweetener has led to various emerging applications and innovations:

- Functional Beverages: Monk fruit sweetener is being incorporated into functional beverages, such as enhanced waters, wellness shots, and sports drinks, to provide natural sweetness without added sugars.
- Plant-Based Foods: Monk fruit sweetener is a popular choice for sweetening plant-based and vegan products, including non-dairy yogurts, cheeses, and meat alternatives.
- Snack Foods: Monk fruit sweetener is being used to create healthier alternatives in the snack food sector, such as low-sugar energy bars, fruit snacks, and baked chips.
- Condiments and Sauces: Innovative applications include using monk fruit sweetener to create low-sugar ketchups, BBQ sauces, and dressings that cater to health-conscious consumers.

Projected growth of the monk fruit sweetener market:

The global sweetener market is experiencing a shift towards healthier alternatives, driving the growth of monk fruit sweetener. While I don't have access to real-time data, as of my last update in September 2021, the monk fruit sweetener market was projected to witness substantial growth due to increasing consumer demand for natural, low-calorie sweeteners. Factors contributing to the projected growth include:

- Health Awareness: As consumers become more health-conscious, the demand for reduced-sugar and zero-calorie sweeteners like monk fruit sweetener continues to rise.
- Diverse Applications: Monk fruit sweetener's versatility allows it to be used in a wide range of food and beverage products, catering to various dietary preferences.
- Clean Label Trend: The clean label movement, which emphasizes simple and natural ingredients, aligns well with monk fruit sweetener's natural origin.
- Regulatory Approvals: As monk fruit sweetener gains regulatory approvals in different countries, it becomes more accessible to a global market.
- Innovation: Continuous innovation in product formulations and applications expands the reach of monk fruit sweetener, attracting consumers looking for healthier options.
- Functional Foods: The integration of monk fruit sweetener into functional foods and beverages further contributes to its market growth.

While market projections indicate a positive trajectory for monk fruit sweetener, it's important to note that market dynamics can change based on various factors, including consumer preferences, technological advancements, and regulatory changes. For the most up-to-date insights, consulting recent market reports and industry analyses is recommended

CHAPTER TWELVE

Monk Fruit Sweetener:
Fact vs. Fiction

Addressing myths and misconceptions surrounding monk fruit sweetener:

- Myth: Monk Fruit Sweetener is Artificial: Monk fruit sweetener is a natural sweetener derived from the monk fruit plant. It is not an artificial sweetener like aspartame or sucralose.
- Myth: Monk Fruit Sweetener Contains Hidden Sugars: Monk fruit sweetener gets its sweetness from natural compounds called mogrosides, which are not sugars. It has no impact on blood sugar levels.
- Myth: Monk Fruit Sweetener Causes Health Issues: Monk fruit sweetener is generally recognized as safe (GRAS) by regulatory agencies like the FDA when used in moderation. It does not cause health issues when consumed as part of a balanced diet.
- Myth: Monk Fruit Sweetener is Bitter: While some monk fruit sweeteners might have a slightly bitter aftertaste, high-quality products go through a purification process to minimize bitterness.

Clarifying rumors about its production process and health implications:

- Rumor: Monk Fruit Sweetener Contains Additives: Quality monk fruit sweeteners contain only monk fruit extract and a natural carrier (like erythritol). Be sure to read ingredient labels to identify any additives.
- Rumor: Monk Fruit Sweetener Harms Gut Bacteria: Research on the impact of monk fruit on gut bacteria is limited, but it is not expected to have a significant negative impact when consumed in moderation.
- Rumor: Monk Fruit Sweetener Causes Allergies: True allergies to monk fruit are rare. However, sensitivities might occur due to other components in the product.

Reliable sources for accurate information about monk fruit sweetener:

- Regulatory Agencies: Check official websites of regulatory agencies like the FDA, EFSA (European Food Safety Authority), and other local health authorities for information on approved sweeteners and their safety.
- Scientific Journals: Peer-reviewed scientific journals publish research studies on monk fruit sweetener's safety, health effects, and production process.
- Reputable Health Organizations: Websites of respected health organizations like Mayo Clinic, American Heart Association, and Diabetes Association often provide accurate information on sweeteners.
- Manufacturer Websites: Reputable monk fruit sweetener manufacturers provide detailed

information about their products, including production methods, quality control, and health implications.

- Nutrition Experts and Dietitians: Registered dietitians and nutrition experts can provide evidence-based information on sweeteners, including monk fruit.
- Academic Institutions: University websites and research centers may offer insights into the latest studies on sweeteners, including monk fruit.

It's important to critically evaluate sources and ensure that the information comes from credible, reliable, and unbiased sources. Misinformation can spread easily, so rely on well-established and trustworthy sources when seeking accurate information about monk fruit sweetener and other food-related topics.

CHAPTER THIRTEEN

Monk Fruit Sweetener Recipes

Refreshing Lemon Mint Iced Tea
Description of the Meal:

Beat the heat with this incredibly refreshing and invigorating iced tea that's sweetened with monk fruit and garnished with zesty lemon slices and fragrant mint leaves. This delightful drink is a perfect balance of flavors, making it a go-to option for hot summer days or any time you need a revitalizing pick-me-up.

Ingredients:

- 4 cups of water
- 4 tea bags (black or green tea)
- 1 lemon, sliced
- A handful of fresh mint leaves
- 1 tablespoon monk fruit sweetener (adjust to taste)
- Ice cubes

Instructions:

- Boil the water and steep the tea bags in it for about 5-7 minutes. Remove the tea bags and allow the tea to cool to room temperature.
- Once the tea has cooled, refrigerate it for at least an hour.
- To serve, fill glasses with ice cubes and pour the

chilled tea over the ice.
- Add lemon slices and mint leaves to each glass.
- Sweeten the tea with monk fruit sweetener, adjusting to your preferred level of sweetness.
- Stir well and enjoy the refreshing blend of flavors!

Nutritional Information:

- Serving Size: 1 glass
- Calories: 10
- Total Fat: 0g
- Sodium: 5mg
- Total Carbohydrates: 3g
- Sugars: 0g
- Protein: 0g

Berries And Yogurt Parfait

Description of the Meal:

Indulge in the delightful medley of flavors and textures in this layered Greek yogurt parfait. Each spoonful is a burst of goodness, with creamy yogurt, juicy mixed berries, crunchy granola, and a drizzle of luscious monk fruit syrup. This parfait is not only visually appealing but also a harmonious blend of sweet and tangy tastes that will satisfy your cravings.

Ingredients:

- 1 cup Greek yogurt
- 1/2 cup mixed berries (strawberries, blueberries, raspberries)
- 1/4 cup granola
- 2 tablespoons monk fruit syrup
- Fresh mint leaves for garnish (optional)

Instructions:

- In a glass or bowl, start by adding a spoonful of Greek yogurt as the first layer.
- Top the yogurt with a handful of mixed berries, creating the second layer.
- Sprinkle a layer of granola over the berries, adding a satisfying crunch.
- Drizzle the monk fruit syrup over the granola, allowing it to infuse sweetness throughout the layers.
- Repeat the layers as desired, finishing with a drizzle of syrup on top.
- Garnish with fresh mint leaves for an extra touch of freshness and color.
- Grab a spoon and dive into the harmonious blend of flavors and textures.

Nutritional Information:

- Serving Size: 1 parfait
- Calories: 220
- Total Fat: 5g
- Sodium: 60mg
- Total Carbohydrates: 35g
- Sugars: 12g
- Protein: 12g

Creamy Almond Milk Oatmeal Bowl

Description of the Meal:

Start your day off right with a bowl of creamy oatmeal cooked to perfection in almond milk. This comforting breakfast is both hearty and wholesome. Topped with sliced bananas, chopped nuts, and a sprinkle of monk fruit and cinnamon, it's a symphony of flavors and textures that will fuel your morning.

Ingredients:

- 1 cup rolled oats
- 2 cups unsweetened almond milk
- 1 ripe banana, sliced
- 2 tablespoons chopped nuts (e.g., almonds, walnuts)
- 1 tablespoon monk fruit sweetener
- ½ teaspoon ground cinnamon

Instructions:

- In a saucepan, bring the almond milk to a gentle simmer.
- Stir in the rolled oats and cook over medium-low heat, stirring occasionally, until the oats are soft and creamy (about 5-7 minutes).
- Remove from heat and stir in the monk fruit sweetener.
- Transfer the oatmeal to a bowl and top with sliced bananas and chopped nuts.
- Sprinkle ground cinnamon over the top for an extra layer of warmth and flavor.
- Grab a spoon and savor the comfort and nourishment of this creamy oatmeal bowl.

Nutritional Information:

- Serving Size: 1 bowl
- Calories: 300
- Total Fat: 10g
- Sodium: 150mg
- Total Carbohydrates: 48g

- Sugars: 8g
- Protein: 8g

Monk Fruit-Glazed Grilled Salmon

Description of the Meal:

Elevate your dinner game with this grilled salmon fillet that's been brushed with a mouthwatering monk fruit glaze. Infused with the flavors of ginger, garlic, and soy sauce, this dish strikes a perfect balance between sweet and savory. Fire up the grill and get ready to enjoy a seafood masterpiece.

Ingredients:

- 2 salmon fillets
- 2 tablespoons monk fruit sweetener
- 1 tablespoon soy sauce
- 1 teaspoon grated ginger
- 2 cloves garlic, minced
- Salt and pepper to taste

Instructions:

- Preheat the grill to medium-high heat.
- In a bowl, mix together the monk fruit sweetener, soy sauce, grated ginger, minced garlic, salt, and pepper to create the glaze.
- Brush the glaze over both sides of the salmon fillets.
- Place the salmon on the grill and cook for about 4-5 minutes on each side, or until the salmon flakes easily with a fork.
- Remove from the grill and serve with your favorite side dishes.

Nutritional Information:

- Serving Size: 1 salmon fillet
- Calories: 300
- Total Fat: 15g
- Sodium: 400mg
- Total Carbohydrates: 8g
- Sugars: 2g
- Protein: 30g

Monk Fruit-Sweetened Zucchini Muffins

Description of the Meal:

Satisfy your cravings with these moist zucchini muffins that have a touch of monk fruit sweetness. Perfect for breakfast or a snack, these treats are a great way to sneak in some veggies. The combination of flavors and the tender crumb make them an irresistible choice.

Ingredients:

- 1 ½ cups all-purpose flour
- ½ cup monk fruit sweetener
- 1 teaspoon baking powder
- ½ teaspoon baking soda
- ½ teaspoon ground cinnamon
- ¼ teaspoon salt
- 1 cup grated zucchini, squeezed to remove excess moisture
- ½ cup unsweetened applesauce
- ¼ cup vegetable oil
- 1 large egg
- 1 teaspoon vanilla extract

Instructions:

- Preheat the oven to 350°F (175°C) and line a muffin tin with paper liners.
- In a bowl, whisk together the flour, monk fruit sweetener, baking powder, baking soda, cinnamon, and salt.
- In another bowl, combine the grated zucchini, applesauce, vegetable oil, egg, and vanilla extract.
- Gradually add the wet ingredients to the dry ingredients, stirring until just combined.
- Divide the batter evenly among the muffin cups, filling each about 2/3 full.
- Bake for 18-20 minutes, or until a toothpick inserted into the center of a muffin comes out clean.
- Allow the muffins to cool in the tin for a few minutes before transferring to a wire rack to cool completely.

Nutritional Information:

- Serving Size: 1 muffin
- Calories: 120
- Total Fat: 6g
- Sodium: 120mg
- Total Carbohydrates: 15g
- Sugars: 3g
- Protein: 2g

Tangy Monk Fruit Barbecue Sauce

Description of the Meal:

Elevate your grilling experience with this tangy and smoky barbecue sauce that's been sweetened with monk fruit. The rich flavors of this sauce, combined with the sweetness of monk fruit, create a delectable balance that's perfect for marinating meats or using as a dipping sauce. Get ready to impress your taste buds!

Ingredients:

- 1 cup tomato ketchup
- ¼ cup apple cider vinegar
- ¼ cup soy sauce
- 2 tablespoons monk fruit sweetener
- 1 tablespoon Dijon mustard
- 1 teaspoon smoked paprika
- ½ teaspoon garlic powder
- ½ teaspoon onion powder
- ¼ teaspoon black pepper

Instructions:

- In a saucepan, combine all the ingredients.
- Bring the mixture to a simmer over medium heat, stirring to combine.
- Reduce the heat to low and let the sauce simmer for about 15-20 minutes, stirring occasionally.
- Once the sauce has thickened and the flavors have melded together, remove from heat and let it cool.
- Use the barbecue sauce to marinate your favorite meats before grilling or serve it as a dipping sauce.

Nutritional Information:

- Serving Size: 2 tablespoons
- Calories: 20
- Total Fat: 0g
- Sodium: 300mg
- Total Carbohydrates: 5g
- Sugars: 1g
- Protein: 1g

Chocolate Avocado Pudding Delight

Description of the Meal:

Indulge in a guilt-free treat with this creamy chocolate pudding that's crafted from ripe avocados and sweetened with monk fruit. The rich, velvety texture of the avocado blends harmoniously with the decadent chocolate flavor, creating a dessert that's both satisfying and nourishing. Topped with a burst of fresh berries and shaved dark chocolate, it's a symphony of tastes and textures that will satisfy your sweet tooth.

Ingredients:

- 2 ripe avocados, peeled and pitted
- ¼ cup unsweetened cocoa powder
- ¼ cup monk fruit sweetener
- ¼ cup almond milk
- 1 teaspoon vanilla extract
- Fresh berries for topping (e.g., strawberries, raspberries)
- Shaved dark chocolate for garnish

Instructions:

- In a food processor, blend the ripe avocados, cocoa powder, monk fruit sweetener, almond milk, and vanilla extract until smooth and creamy.
- Taste and adjust sweetness if needed by adding more monk fruit sweetener.
- Divide the pudding into serving cups or bowls.
- Top with fresh berries and a sprinkle of shaved dark chocolate.
- Refrigerate for about 1 hour before serving to

allow the flavors to meld.

Nutritional Information:

- Serving Size: 1 serving
- Calories: 180
- Total Fat: 15g
- Sodium: 10mg
- Total Carbohydrates: 15g
- Sugars: 2g
- Protein: 3g

Monk Fruit-Enhanced Salad Dressing

Description of the Meal:

Elevate your salads with this light and flavorful salad dressing that features monk fruit as the sweetener. This dressing perfectly balances tanginess and sweetness, making it an ideal complement to a fresh and vibrant salad. It's an excellent way to enjoy a guilt-free burst of flavors.

Ingredients:

- ¼ cup olive oil
- 2 tablespoons balsamic vinegar
- 1 teaspoon Dijon mustard
- ½ teaspoon monk fruit sweetener
- Salt and pepper to taste

Instructions:

- In a small bowl, whisk together the olive oil, balsamic vinegar, Dijon mustard, and monk fruit sweetener until well combined.
- Season with salt and pepper to taste.
- Drizzle the dressing over your favorite salad just before serving.

- Toss the salad to coat the ingredients evenly with the dressing.

Nutritional Information:

- Serving Size: 2 tablespoons
- Calories: 90
- Total Fat: 9g
- Sodium: 80mg
- Total Carbohydrates: 2g
- Sugars: 1g
- Protein: 0g

Monk Fruit Blueberry Almond Pancakes

Description of the Meal:

Start your morning on a sweet note with these fluffy blueberry pancakes made with almond flour and sweetened with monk fruit. The combination of nutty almond flavor and the burst of blueberries creates a pancake experience that's both satisfying and wholesome. Serve these delightful pancakes with sugar-free syrup for a guilt-free breakfast treat.

Ingredients:

- 1 cup almond flour
- 2 tablespoons monk fruit sweetener
- 1 teaspoon baking powder
- ¼ teaspoon salt
- 2 large eggs
- ¼ cup unsweetened almond milk
- ½ teaspoon vanilla extract
- ½ cup fresh blueberries

Instructions:

- In a bowl, whisk together the almond flour, monk fruit sweetener, baking powder, and salt.
- In another bowl, beat the eggs, then add the almond milk and vanilla extract. Mix well.
- Combine the wet and dry ingredients, stirring until just combined.
- Gently fold in the fresh blueberries.
- Heat a non-stick skillet over medium heat and lightly grease it.
- Pour a ladleful of batter onto the skillet to form a pancake.
- Cook until bubbles form on the surface, then flip and cook the other side until golden brown.
- Repeat with the remaining batter.

Nutritional Information:

- Serving Size: 2 pancakes
- Calories: 220
- Total Fat: 18g
- Sodium: 220mg
- Total Carbohydrates: 9g
- Sugars: 2g
- Protein: 8g

Lemon-Glazed Grilled Chicken With Roasted Vegetables

Description of the Meal:

Savor the combination of flavors in this grilled chicken dish with a zesty lemon glaze sweetened by monk fruit. The juicy chicken breasts are elevated with a tangy and slightly sweet glaze, creating a perfect balance of tastes. Accompanied by a side of roasted vegetables, this meal is a wholesome and satisfying option for lunch or dinner.

Ingredients:

- 2 boneless, skinless chicken breasts
- Zest and juice of 1 lemon
- 2 tablespoons monk fruit sweetener
- 2 cloves garlic, minced
- Salt and pepper to taste
- Assorted vegetables for roasting (e.g., bell peppers, zucchini, carrots)
- Olive oil for roasting

Instructions:

- In a bowl, whisk together the lemon zest, lemon juice, monk fruit sweetener, minced garlic, salt, and pepper to create the glaze.
- Brush the glaze over both sides of the chicken breasts.
- Preheat the grill to medium-high heat.
- Grill the chicken breasts for about 6-7 minutes on each side, or until the internal temperature reaches 165°F (74°C).
- While the chicken is grilling, toss the assorted vegetables with olive oil, salt, and pepper.
- Roast the vegetables in the oven at 400°F (200°C) until they are tender and slightly caramelized.
- Serve the grilled chicken with the roasted vegetables on the side.

Nutritional Information:

- Serving Size: 1 chicken breast with vegetables
- Calories: 350
- Total Fat: 12g
- Sodium: 350mg

- Total Carbohydrates: 20g
- Sugars: 8g
- Protein: 40g

Coconut Chia Pudding Parfait

Description of the Meal:

Delight in the delightful textures and flavors of this coconut chia pudding parfait. Chia seeds are soaked in creamy coconut milk and monk fruit sweetener, resulting in a pudding that's both indulgent and nourishing. Topped with toasted coconut flakes and chopped nuts, each spoonful is a tropical treat that offers a perfect balance of richness and crunch.

Ingredients:

- ¼ cup chia seeds
- 1 cup coconut milk (canned or carton)
- 1 tablespoon monk fruit sweetener
- 2 tablespoons toasted coconut flakes
- 2 tablespoons chopped nuts (e.g., almonds, cashews)

Instructions:

- In a bowl, combine the chia seeds, coconut milk, and monk fruit sweetener.
- Stir well to ensure the chia seeds are evenly distributed in the milk.
- Cover the bowl and refrigerate for at least 4 hours or overnight, allowing the chia seeds to absorb the liquid and create a pudding-like consistency.
- Before serving, give the chia pudding a good stir.
- Spoon the chia pudding into serving glasses and

top with toasted coconut flakes and chopped nuts.
- Enjoy the layers of flavors and textures in this coconut chia pudding parfait.

Nutritional Information:

- Serving Size: 1 parfait
- Calories: 300
- Total Fat: 25g
- Sodium: 20mg
- Total Carbohydrates: 14g
- Sugars: 1g
- Protein: 7g

Monk Fruit Sweetened Cold Brew Coffee

Description of the Meal:

Stay refreshed and energized with this cold brew coffee that's been sweetened with monk fruit syrup and enhanced with a splash of almond milk. Served over ice, this coffee is a smooth and invigorating pick-me-up that offers a balance of rich coffee flavor and subtle sweetness.

Ingredients:

- 1 cup cold brew coffee
- 1 tablespoon monk fruit syrup
- Splash of almond milk
- Ice cubes

Instructions:

- Fill a glass with ice cubes.
- Pour the cold brew coffee over the ice.
- Add the monk fruit syrup and a splash of almond milk.
- Stir well to combine and chill the coffee.

- Sip and enjoy the revitalizing flavors of this monk fruit sweetened cold brew coffee.

Nutritional Information:

- Serving Size: 1 glass
- Calories: 10
- Total Fat: 0g
- Sodium: 5mg
- Total Carbohydrates: 2g
- Sugars: 0g
- Protein: 0g

Monk Fruit Sweetened Stir-Fried Vegetables With Cauliflower Rice

Description of the Meal:

Indulge in a burst of colors and flavors with this colorful stir-fried vegetables and cauliflower rice dish. The savory sauce, sweetened with monk fruit, beautifully coats the vibrant vegetables and cauliflower rice. Each bite is a symphony of tastes and textures, creating a wholesome and satisfying meal.

Ingredients:

- 2 cups mixed vegetables (bell peppers, carrots, broccoli, snap peas, etc.)
- 2 cups cauliflower rice
- 2 tablespoons olive oil
- 2 tablespoons soy sauce
- 1 tablespoon monk fruit sweetener
- 1 teaspoon sesame oil
- 1 teaspoon minced garlic
- ½ teaspoon grated ginger

- Salt and pepper to taste

Instructions:

- Heat olive oil in a large skillet or wok over medium-high heat.
- Add the minced garlic and grated ginger, and stir-fry for about 30 seconds.
- Add the mixed vegetables and stir-fry for 3-4 minutes, until they are tender-crisp.
- Push the vegetables to the side of the skillet and add the cauliflower rice. Cook for an additional 2-3 minutes.
- In a bowl, whisk together the soy sauce, monk fruit sweetener, and sesame oil.
- Pour the sauce over the vegetables and cauliflower rice. Stir to combine and coat evenly.
- Season with salt and pepper to taste.
- Serve the stir-fried vegetables and cauliflower rice hot, enjoying the delightful blend of flavors.

Nutritional Information:

- Serving Size: 1 plate
- Calories: 200
- Total Fat: 12g
- Sodium: 700mg
- Total Carbohydrates: 18g
- Sugars: 8g
- Protein: 6g

Apple Cinnamon Nutty Energy Bites

Description of the Meal:

Fuel your day with these nutty energy bites that

are bursting with the flavors of oats, chopped apples, cinnamon, and monk fruit sweetness. These bites are a perfect combination of nutrients and taste, making them a convenient and satisfying snack option for those on the go.

Ingredients:

- 1 cup rolled oats
- ½ cup chopped apples
- ¼ cup almond butter
- ¼ cup monk fruit sweetener
- 1 teaspoon ground cinnamon
- ½ teaspoon vanilla extract
- Pinch of salt

Instructions:

- In a bowl, combine the rolled oats, chopped apples, almond butter, monk fruit sweetener, ground cinnamon, vanilla extract, and a pinch of salt.
- Mix well until the ingredients come together.
- Using your hands, roll small portions of the mixture into bite-sized balls.
- Place the energy bites on a plate or tray lined with parchment paper.
- Refrigerate the bites for at least 30 minutes to firm up.
- Enjoy these nutty energy bites as a quick and satisfying snack.

Nutritional Information:

- Serving Size: 2 energy bites
- Calories: 150
- Total Fat: 7g
- Sodium: 30mg
- Total Carbohydrates: 20g

- Sugars: 5g
- Protein: 4g

Monk Fruit Sweetened Raspberry Sorbet

Description of the Meal:

Savor the refreshing raspberry sorbet that's made without added sugar and sweetened exclusively with monk fruit. This frozen treat is a burst of natural sweetness and tanginess that's perfect for cooling down on warm days. Each spoonful is a delightful way to indulge your taste buds without the guilt.

Ingredients:

- 3 cups fresh raspberries
- ¼ cup monk fruit sweetener
- 1 tablespoon lemon juice

Instructions:

- Place the fresh raspberries in a blender or food processor.
- Add the monk fruit sweetener and lemon juice to the raspberries.
- Blend until the mixture is smooth and well combined.
- Pour the raspberry mixture into a freezer-safe container.
- Cover the container and freeze the sorbet for at least 4 hours, or until it's firm.
- When ready to serve, let the sorbet sit at room temperature for a few minutes to soften slightly before scooping.

Nutritional Information:

- Serving Size: 1 scoop
- Calories: 40
- Total Fat: 1g
- Sodium: 0mg
- Total Carbohydrates: 9g
- Sugars: 4g
- Protein: 1g

CHAPTER FOURTEEN

Testimonials and Success Stories

Real-life experiences of individuals who have embraced monk fruit sweetener:

Monk fruit sweetener has made a positive impact on the lives of many individuals who have chosen to incorporate it into their diets. Here are some real-life experiences:

1. Weight Loss and Lifestyle Change:

Sarah, a 35-year-old, shared how using monk fruit sweetener played a pivotal role in her weight loss journey. Struggling with a sweet tooth, she found traditional sugars contributed to her calorie intake. Switching to monk fruit sweetener allowed her to enjoy sweetness without the guilt. Over time, Sarah lost weight and found it easier to manage her overall calorie intake.

2. Blood Sugar Management:

David, a 45-year-old with type 2 diabetes, noticed significant improvements in his blood sugar levels after adopting monk fruit sweetener. He replaced sugar in his morning coffee and dessert recipes with monk fruit sweetener. With regular monitoring and the support of his healthcare team, David experienced more stable blood sugar readings, reducing his reliance on insulin.

3. Healthier Baking and Cooking:

Emma, a mother of two, was determined to provide healthier options for her family's favorite treats. She began experimenting with monk fruit sweetener in her baking and cooking. Not only did her family enjoy the results, but they also felt better knowing they were consuming fewer empty calories and refined sugars.

4. Reduced Sugar Cravings:

John, a fitness enthusiast, struggled with sugar cravings that interfered with his diet goals. Incorporating monk fruit sweetener into his post-workout shakes and protein bars allowed him to satisfy his cravings without consuming excess calories. He found that over time, his cravings for sugary snacks decreased.

5. Balanced Diabetic Diet:

Rebecca, diagnosed with gestational diabetes during pregnancy, sought alternatives to manage her blood sugar levels while still enjoying her meals. With her doctor's guidance, she integrated monk fruit sweetener into her diet. It helped her maintain steady blood sugar levels and provided the sweetness she craved without negatively affecting her health.

It's important to note that individual experiences can vary. While monk fruit sweetener has shown positive outcomes for some individuals, results depend on various factors, including overall diet, lifestyle, health conditions, and personal preferences. Consulting a healthcare professional before making dietary changes, especially for individuals with diabetes or other health conditions, is recommended to ensure that monk fruit sweetener aligns with individual needs and goals.

CHAPTER FIFTEEN

Embracing a Healthier Sweetener Choice

Summary of Benefits and Practical Uses of Monk Fruit Sweetener:

Monk fruit sweetener is a natural, zero-calorie sweetener derived from the monk fruit plant. Its benefits and practical uses make it an attractive choice for health-conscious individuals seeking to reduce sugar intake and achieve a balanced lifestyle. Here are some key points:

Benefits:

- Zero Calories: Monk fruit sweetener provides sweetness without adding calories, making it a valuable tool for weight management and calorie-conscious diets.
- Low Glycemic Impact: It doesn't cause significant spikes in blood sugar levels, making it suitable for individuals with diabetes and those monitoring blood sugar.
- Natural Origin: Monk fruit sweetener is derived from a fruit and often minimally processed, appealing to those seeking natural alternatives.
- Versatility: It can be used in a variety of recipes, including beverages, desserts, sauces, and more.
- Clean Label: Monk fruit sweetener aligns with

clean label trends, as it contains few ingredients and no artificial additives.

Practical Uses:

- Sweetening Beverages: Add monk fruit sweetener to coffee, tea, smoothies, and other beverages for a touch of sweetness.
- Baking and Cooking: Substitute sugar with monk fruit sweetener in recipes for baked goods, sauces, dressings, and more.
- Low-Sugar Treats: Create guilt-free desserts and snacks by incorporating monk fruit sweetener into recipes.
- Mindful Eating: Use it to foster mindful eating habits by enjoying sweet flavors without the drawbacks of excess sugar.
- Special Diets: Monk fruit sweetener is suitable for keto, paleo, diabetic, and low-carb diets.

Making Informed Decisions for Dietary Preferences:

As consumers, making informed decisions about the foods and sweeteners we choose is essential. Monk fruit sweetener offers a healthier alternative to traditional sugars and artificial sweeteners. When considering its use, it's important to:

- Research: Learn about monk fruit sweetener's benefits, usage, and potential health implications from reputable sources.
- Consult Professionals: If you have specific health concerns or dietary restrictions, consult healthcare professionals or registered dietitians for personalized guidance.
- Read Labels: When purchasing monk fruit

sweetener products, read ingredient labels to ensure you're getting a quality product with minimal additives.

- Experiment: Experiment with monk fruit sweetener in recipes to find the right balance of sweetness and taste for your preferences.

Emphasizing the Role of Monk Fruit Sweetener in Fostering a Balanced Lifestyle:

Monk fruit sweetener fits seamlessly into a balanced lifestyle by allowing you to enjoy sweetness while making healthier choices. It offers the opportunity to satisfy cravings without compromising your goals. By incorporating monk fruit sweetener into your diet, you can:

- Reduce Sugar Intake: Enjoy sweetness without the negative impacts of excessive sugar consumption on weight, blood sugar, and overall health.
- Support Weight Management: Substitute traditional sugars with monk fruit sweetener to reduce calorie intake and aid in weight loss or maintenance.
- Mindful Eating: Foster mindful eating by savoring flavors and enjoying treats in moderation, thanks to the guilt-free sweetness provided by monk fruit.
- Diverse Applications: Its versatility in various recipes empowers you to create a wide range of delicious and health-conscious dishes.

Ultimately, monk fruit sweetener empowers you to take control of your dietary choices, supporting your journey toward a balanced and health-conscious lifestyle. By making informed decisions and incorporating monk fruit sweetener thoughtfully, you can enjoy sweetness without compromise and enhance your overall well-being.

CONCLUSION

In conclusion, monk fruit sweetener stands as a remarkable testament to the possibilities of nature's sweetness. Its journey from an ancient medicinal herb to a modern, natural sweetener has brought a myriad of benefits to our tables and lifestyles. As we embrace the evolution of our dietary choices, monk fruit sweetener offers a pathway to healthier living, allowing us to savor the sweetness of life without the drawbacks of excessive sugars. Its zero-calorie nature, low glycemic impact, and versatility in various culinary creations make it a valuable addition to our quest for balanced and mindful consumption.

In an era where wellness and conscious eating are paramount, monk fruit sweetener shines as a symbol of progress and innovation. From kitchens to commercial products, its presence has transformed the way we sweeten our lives. While myths and misconceptions may linger, it's imperative to turn to reliable sources and trusted experts for accurate information.

Let us celebrate the potential of monk fruit sweetener to enhance our daily experiences, making our favorite dishes a little healthier and our indulgences a little smarter. As we savor the sweetness it brings, let's continue to make informed choices, embracing its benefits as part of our journey toward a more balanced, health-conscious lifestyle. Monk fruit sweetener is not just a sweet addition to our diets; it's a testament to our commitment to better living.

Printed in Great Britain
by Amazon

41243159R00042